THINGS TO KNOW ABOUT CHOLESTEROL:

Why Reducing Cholesterol Won't Stop Heart Disease

By

Michael D. Davis

TABLE OF CONTENTS

The production of hormones is facilitated by cholesterol. The synthesis of bile acids requires cholesterol to be present in the body. The cell membranes of every single cell in the body need cholesterol to function correctly. The immune system benefits greatly from cholesterol's presence. Vitamin D is derived from cholesterol in our bodies. When you have a solid grasp of this much-maligned molecule's roles in the body, you'll have a better understanding of the myriad of problems that might arise from the pursuit of ever-lower cholesterol levels.

The most common cause of death is heart disease. On the other hand, traditional treatments for heart disease have been entirely misguided. Science is demonstrating that cholesterol and saturated fat do not play a direct role in the development of heart disease and that the standard recommendation of low-fat diets and statin drugs is contributing to a health crisis of monumental proportions.Sugar (not fat), inflammation, stress, and high-carb diets full of processed foods are some of the true causes of heart disease discussed in The Great Cholesterol Myth. This book exposes the poor science, manipulated research, and corporate greed that have contributed to the perpetuation of the myth that cholesterol causes heart disease.

CHAPTER 1

WHAT IS CHOLESTEROL: Why you ought to have some serious misgivings of LDL as a mark of coronary illness

Cholesterol is a waxy substance. It's not innately "terrible." Your body needs it to fabricate cells and make nutrients and different chemicals. Yet, an excess of cholesterol can represent an issue.

Cholesterol comes from two sources. Your liver makes all the cholesterol you want. The rest of the cholesterol in your body comes from food varieties from creatures. For instance, meat, poultry, and dairy items all contain dietary cholesterol.

Those equivalent food varieties are high in soaked and trans fats. These fats make your liver make more cholesterol than it in any case would. For certain individuals, this additional creation implies they go from an ordinary cholesterol level to one that is undesirable.

A few tropical oils -, for example, palm oil, palm bit oil, and coconut oil - contain soaked fat that can increment terrible cholesterol. These oils are much of the time tracked down in prepared merchandise.
Why cholesterol matters
Cholesterol flows in the blood. As how much cholesterol in your blood increments, so does the gamble on your well-being. Elevated cholesterol adds to

a higher gamble of cardiovascular illnesses, like coronary illness and stroke. That is the reason it's vital to have your cholesterol tried, so you can know your levels.

The two sorts of cholesterol are LDL cholesterol, which is awful, and great HDL. A lot of the terrible kind, or insufficient of the great kind, expands the gamble cholesterol will gradually develop in the internal walls of the courses that feed the heart and mind.

Kind of cholesterol

Cholesterol is moved around the body in the circulation system on proteins called lipoproteins. There are two kinds of lipoprotein: low-thickness lipoprotein (LDL), which is some of the time called "terrible" cholesterol, and high-thickness lipoprotein (HDL), additionally alluded to as "great cholesterol."

A high LDL level is related to an expanded gamble for coronary illness and stroke. LDL transports cholesterol to the veins, and when the LDL level is raised, this cholesterol can collect in the vein walls and add to the development of a plaque. This plaque arrangement, or atherosclerosis, can ultimately make the vessel restricted and decline the bloodstream to the heart (coronary supply route sickness). Assuming the vessel becomes hindered so that blood no longer arrives at the heart or mind, this can bring about chest torment (angina), coronary episodes, or stroke.

HDL represents high-thickness lipoproteins. It is now and again called the "upside" cholesterol since it conveys cholesterol from different pieces of your body back to your liver. Your liver then, at that point, eliminates the cholesterol from your body.

How do I have any idea about what my HDL level is?

A blood test can quantify your cholesterol levels, including HDL. When and how frequently you ought to get this test relies upon your age, risk elements, and family ancestry. The overall proposals are:

For individuals who are age 19 or more youthful:

• The principal test ought to be between ages 9 to 11
• Kids ought to have the test once more like clockwork
• A few kids might have this test beginning at age 2 if there is a family background of high blood cholesterol, coronary episode, or stroke

For individuals who are age 20 or more established:

• More youthful grown-ups ought to have the test like clockwork
• Men ages 45 to 65 and ladies ages 55 to 65 ought to have it each 1 to 2 years

What should my HDL even out be?

With HDL cholesterol, larger numbers are better, because a high HDL level can bring down your gamble for coronary vein infection and stroke. How high your HDL ought to rely upon your age and sex:

Group Healthy HDL Level

Age 19 or younger More than 45mg/dl

Men age 20 or older More than 40mg/dl

Ladies age 20 or older with More than 50mg/dl

How might I raise my HDL level?

If your HDL level is excessively low, your way of life changes might help. These progressions may likewise assist with forestalling different infections, and cheer you up by and large:

• Eat a solid eating routine. To raise your HDL level, you want to eat great fats rather than terrible fats. This implies restricting immersed fats, which incorporate full-fat milk and cheddar, high-fat meats like frankfurter and bacon, and food sources made with margarine, grease, and shortening. You ought to likewise keep away from trans fats, which might be in certain margarine, broiled food varieties, and handled food sources like prepared merchandise. All things being equal, eat unsaturated fats, which are found in avocado, vegetable oils like olive oil, and nuts. Limit starches, particularly sugar. Likewise attempt to eat more food sources normally high in fiber, like oats and beans.

• Remain at a solid weight. You can support your HDL level by getting in shape, particularly assuming you have loads of fat around your midriff.

• Work out. Getting standard activity can raise your HDL level, as well as lower your LDL. You ought to attempt to complete 30 minutes of moderate to overwhelming high-impact practice on the vast majority of days.

• Keep away from cigarettes. Smoking and openness to second-hand smoke can bring down your HDL level. On the off chance that you are a smoker, ask your medical services supplier for help in tracking down the most effective way for you to stop. You ought to likewise attempt to keep away from recycled smoke.
• Limit liquor. Moderate liquor might bring down your HDL level, albeit more investigations are expected to affirm that. What we can be sure of is that an excessive amount of liquor can make you put on weight, and that brings down your HDL level.
Some cholesterol medications, including specific statins, can raise your HDL level, as well as bring down your LDL level. Medical services suppliers don't generally endorse meds just to raise HDL. In any case, on the off chance that you have a low HDL and high LDL level, you could require medication.
What else can influence my HDL even out?
Taking specific drugs can bring down HDL levels in certain individuals. They include:
• Beta blockers, a sort of circulatory strain medication
• Anabolic steroids, including testosterone, a male chemical
• Progestins, which are female chemicals that are in some conception prevention pills and chemical substitution treatment
• Benzodiazepines, tranquilizers that are frequently utilized for nervousness and sleep deprivation

If you are taking one of these and you have an exceptionally low HDL level, inquire as to whether you ought to keep on taking them.

Diabetes can likewise bring down your HDL level, so that gives you one more motivation to deal with your diabetes.

What is LDL

LDL represents low-thickness lipoprotein. It's a kind of lipoprotein tracked down in your blood. LDL is the "awful cholesterol" because a lot of it in your blood can add to plaque development in your corridors. Food sources with high measures of immersed fat (like full-fat dairy and red meat) can raise your LDL. A heart-solid eating routine, practice, and stopping tobacco use can assist with bringing down your LDL. For the vast majority, a typical LDL level is under 100 mg/dL. The vast majority use "LDL" and "LDL cholesterol" conversely. LDL cholesterol has gained notoriety for being the "terrible cholesterol." However, that is just important for the story. LDL cholesterol itself isn't awful. That is because cholesterol carries out significant roles in your body. Notwithstanding, when you have a lot of LDL cholesterol, that is the point at which you can run into issues.

An abundance of LDL cholesterol adds to plaque development (atherosclerosis) in your corridors. This plague develop may prompt:

- Coronary conduit sickness.
- Cerebrovascular sickness.
- Fringe conduit sickness.
- Aortic aneurysm

Therefore, medical care suppliers urge you to have a sound degree of LDL cholesterol.

What is the LDL cholesterol typical reach?

Most grown-ups ought to keep their LDL under 100 milligrams for each decilitre (mg/dL). If you have a background marked by atherosclerosis, your LDL ought to be under 70 mg/dL.

What is a terrible level for LDL?

An LDL level over 100 mg/dL raises your gamble of cardiovascular illness. Medical care suppliers utilize the accompanying classifications to depict your LDL cholesterol level:

- Typical: Under 100 mg/dL.
- Close ideal: 100 - 129 mg/dL.
- Marginal high: 130 - 159 mg/dL.
- High: 160 - 189 mg/dL.
- Exceptionally high: 190 mg/dL or higher.

Medical care suppliers check your cholesterol levels through a basic blood test called a lipid board. At the point when you accept your outcomes, it's essential to converse with your supplier about what your cholesterol number means. These incorporate two of your LDL and your HDL cholesterol. HDL is the "great cholesterol" that helps eliminate additional cholesterol from your blood.

For the most part, medical services suppliers support higher HDL cholesterol levels (in a perfect world over 60) and lower LDL cholesterol levels to lessen your cardiovascular illness risk. Assuming that your LDL is too high and your HDL is too low, your supplier might suggest a way of life changes and additional meds to get your cholesterol numbers into the sound reach.

What causes high LDL cholesterol?

Many variables can raise your LDL level. The elements you have some command over include:

• What you eat. Food sources like greasy meats, full-fat dairy items, bread kitchens, and quick food varieties are hurtful to your cholesterol levels. That is because they contain high measures of soaked fat and, at times, trans fat. These two sorts of fats raise your LDL cholesterol.

• Your body loads. Having overweight/corpulence can raise your LDL cholesterol.

• Smoking or utilizing tobacco items. Tobacco use (counting smokeless tobacco and vaping) brings down your HDL level. You want a sound measure of HDL cholesterol to dispose of additional LDL cholesterol from your blood. Thus, by lessening your HDL level, tobacco use prompts a raised LDL level.

Factors you have zero control over include:

• Age. As you progress in years, your cholesterol levels normally go up.

• Sex allocated upon entering the world. Individuals allocated females upon entering the world (AFAB) regularly have higher LDL levels after menopause.

• Your qualities. If your nearby natural relatives have elevated cholesterol, you might confront a higher gamble, as well.

What food sources cause high LDL cholesterol?

Food sources that contain high measures of immersed fat are the greatest guilty parties in raising your LDL cholesterol. Such food sources include:

• Bread kitchen things, similar to doughnuts, treats, and cake.

• Full-fat dairy items, similar to entire milk, cheddar, and margarine.

• Red meats, similar to steak, ribs, pork slashes, and ground beef
hamburger.

• Handled meats, similar to bacon, franks, and hotdog.

• Broiled food sources, similar to French fries and seared chicken.

How would I bring down my LDL cholesterol?

There's a ton you can do to bring down your LDL cholesterol. For some individuals, beginning with a way of life changes can have a major effect. Here are a few changes you can make:

• Follow a heart-sound eating regimen. Research shows the Mediterranean eating regimen can bring down your gamble for cardiovascular sickness. This diet urges you to practice good eating habits fats (from sources like olive oil and nuts) and keep away from unfortunate fats (like immersed fat).

• Stay away from tobacco use. Assuming that you smoke, vape or utilize any tobacco items presently is the time to stop. Ask your supplier for assets to help.

• Get more activity. Go for the gold of high-impact practice each day no less than five days per week. Begin slow (only five or 10 minutes all at once) and continuously move gradually up. Converse with your medical services supplier before starting another activity plan or making changes to your old daily schedule.

• Keep a weight that is good for you. Converse with your supplier about what your ideal weight territory ought to be.

• Track down methodologies to bring down your pressure. Being under pressure for quite a while may raise your LDL and lessen your HDL. Methods like yoga or profound breathing activities might assist you with overseeing pressure in your routine.

Your medical care supplier may likewise endorse a prescription to bring down your LDL cholesterol.

Food sources that can bring down your LDL cholesterol

Research demonstrates the way that solvent fiber can bring down your LDL cholesterol. This type of fiber (roughage) blocks the assimilation of cholesterol in your body. You ought to plan to consume 10 to 25 grams (g) each day. Converse with your medical care supplier or a dietitian about the sum that is ideal for you.

The outline underneath records food sources that you can add to your eating regimen to expand your solvent fibre consumption.

Food Serving size Soluble fibre content

Dark beans 3/4 cup
5.4 g
Lima beans 3/4 cup 5.3 g
Naval force beans 3/4 cup 3.3 g
Pinto beans 3/4 cup 3.2 g
Kidney beans 3/4 cup 2.6 - 3.0 g
Tofu 3/4 cup 2.8 g
Avocado 1/2 fruit 2.1 g
Chickpeas 3/4 cup 2.1 g
Brussels sprouts 1/2 cup 2 g
Sweet potato 1/2 cup 1.8 g
Turnips 1/2 cup 1.7 g
Asparagus 1/2 cup 1.7 g
Broccoli 1/2 cup 1.2 - 1.5 g
Cereal (cooked) 3/4 cup 1.4 g
Eggplant 1/2 cup 1.3 g
Carrots 1/2 cup 1.1 - 1.2 g
Apple 1 medium 1.0 g
Beets 1/2 cup .8 g
Banana 1 medium .7 g
Brown rice 1/2 cup .5 g
Conversing with a dietitian can assist you with learning new and innovative ways of integrating these food sources into your everyday dinners.

CHAPTER 2

SUGAR: The genuine evil presence in the diet

With related well-being dangers, for example, stomach harmfulness, diabetes, teeth, liver and neurological harm, raised cholesterol, coronary illness, and connections to malignant growth, it's no big surprise sugar has turned into the evilest of sauces. In any case, before you get on board with the counter sugar fad, you should re-examine removing sugar altogether. As indicated by dietitian and pioneer behind Shift Nourishment, Skye Swanley, taking out sugar totally from your eating routine is certainly not an insightful move, nor is it a solid one.

"We have this win big or bust demeanour with regards to slimming down," Skye says. "All in any case, as a rule disposing of a whole nutrition class out of your eating routine will be more unfavourable to your wellbeing than gainful." Skye's problem with the counter-sugar development is that sugar is being slandered in its structures. In actuality, it's just the handled, refined sorts of sugar that are connected to unexpected problems. At the point when sugar is found in its regular state, for example, the fructose and glucose you find in natural products, going with minerals and fiber inside the natural product aid the sluggish arrival of the sugar.

"Besides the reality, organic product assists give us the energy with filling we run on, they are likewise unbelievably supplement thick so when you kill them from your eating regimen it can have a cost for your wellbeing and nourishment levels."

By and large, this fulfills the desire. Yet, for some, there is an enthusiastic craving to rehash that joy or "high" when it's areas of strength for too even consider standing up to. As you eat more desserts to get that high once more, your body turns out to be more insulin safe. The importance you'll require increasingly more to get similar feels. Graciousness and enslavement are just a single contributor to the issue... We've yet to try and cover the aftereffects of the over-utilization of SUGAR. So while I have you, we should get into that. Here are seven motivations behind why SUGAR is Satan

1. Weight Gain

At the point when your blood glucose levels rise and your body answers by invigorating insulin (this is a characteristic reaction); setting off your body to flip the on change to enact fat (energy) putting away mode. The more predictable you are with your sugar utilization, the more drawn out, and all the more much of the time your body will work in fat-putting-away mode. There are ways of forestalling this, however, and it begins with schooling... Then moves to activity. Assuming you end up on some unacceptable side of, as far as possible your sugar utilization, begin to investigate the glycemia file. This framework positions food varieties (carbs) on a scale from 1 to 100 in light of their impact on glucose levels. Main concern: Make starches (sugars) work for you, and not the reverse way around.

2. Insusceptible Framework Concealment

Sugar admission can smother your safe framework up after utilization. As per Wellbeing Administrations at Columbia College, when you eat 100 grams of sugar, probably as much sugar as you find in a 1-liter jug of pop, your white platelets are 40% less powerful at killing microorganisms. This can disable your safe framework for as long as 5 hours in the wake of eating sugar! Bottom Line: Overutilization of sugar makes you more powerless to ailment and can slow your recuperation cycle if you are as of now debilitated.

3. Type 2 Diabetes

Type 2 diabetes happens because of an absence of insulin creation or expanded protection from insulin. Insulin is a chemical created by the pancreas that takes into consideration the guideline of the take-up of glucose (sugar). It is delivered in light of expanded glucose levels in the blood and considers individual cells to take up glucose from the blood to process it. A high-sugar diet has been connected with an expanded occurrence of Type 2 diabetes because of the connections between high sugar admission and weight. Throughout the long-term abundance of sugar, utilization can make our bodies conceivably quit creating insulin altogether. Difficulties include visual impairment, removal of extremities, misery, neuropathy, sexual brokenness, kidney illness, and dementia. Primary concern: Type 2 Diabetes is a detail you DON'T need on your doctor's report.

4. Coronary illness

In various examinations, an immediate connection has been displayed between expanded sugar utilization and demise from cardiovascular sickness. At the point when insulin levels spike persistently the endothelial coating of the veins becomes harmed which makes aggravation. This constant irritation, combined with hypertension, abundance weight, and unfortunate heart well-being, may ultimately prompt cardiovascular failure. Main concern: Terrible eating routine + (Absence of activity) = An incredible opportunity for coronary illness

5. Irritation in Your Stomach

At the point when your body digests the sugar, it changes the proportion of good microbes to terrible microorganisms in your stomach… And not positively. Terrible microbes flourish off of sugar and can cause various sicknesses since they produce a wide range of hurtful poisons. Other than feeling run down and low energy, the expansion in this harmful microbe can cause yeast contaminations, immune system problems, joint pain, coronary illness, and numerous different afflictions. Primary concern: Recuperate your stomach to accomplish maximal well-being!

6. Retention of Nutrients and Minerals

For the vast majority of us (those functioning out a couple of days out of the week), the utilization of sugar doesn't yield positive well-being and wellness benefits. Taking into account the way that sugar (as a large portion of us know it today) comes up short on sorts of critical supplements, nutrients, or minerals... It's best we simply let it be! Truth be told, an abundance of sugar utilization can thus exhaust the group of zinc, magnesium, potassium, and chromium. Main concern: Sugar in a real sense denies your body the things you want for good well-being.

7. Advances in Disease Cell Development

News reports generally allude to sugar as being "fuel" for malignant growth cells. Furthermore, that is valid — however primarily because sugar is the fuel for all cells in the body. Sugar is a starch, and when you eat any kind of carb (whether it's a natural product or frozen yogurt, or a bagel) your pancreas produces insulin, a chemical that helps convert sugars into energy for your cells. Eating an excessive amount of sugar, however, can make the body insulin safe, meaning it needs to produce increasingly more of the chemical to take care of its business. Quick version, this gooey cycle can likewise deliver to a greater degree a chemical known as insulin-like development factor (IGF), which exploration has displayed to invigorate cell development and hinder cell demise. As such, IGF permits disease to multiply. Disease cells are regularly held within proper limits by the body's consistent turnover — new solid cells develop and awful cells kick the bucket. Main concern: An abundance of IGF blocks the signs for cells to develop typically and bite the dust when now is the ideal time to kick the bucket, so all things being equal they simply develop. So, whenever you're going after your desserts, mull over the thing you're putting inside your body.

Our body is just not intended to deal with this a lot of sugar.

As sugar was initially a valuable product, just found occasionally in ready natural products or periodic honey, our hereditary plan remembered it as a fast and powerful method for getting valuable calories while getting food was the entire day try!

So, our mind became wired to answer sugar very much like it answers drugs like energizers and narcotics, making you need more!

This component is currently working today, and to make things most obviously awful the physiology of our body intensifies the impact since sugar spikes our glucose, and afterward, it crashes it, causing us to ache for more, and that's just the beginning… .and that's only the tip of the iceberg!

This is how we let completely go over our resolve because the motivations of our body become sufficiently able to supersede even the most grounded individual's will.

So how would we get away from this descending twisting? How would we break the endless loop?

The most effective way, as I would see it, is to dispose of the desires. When the body is liberated from the habit, it will be significantly simpler to free the psyche.

However, at that point how would we do that, on the off chance that we cannot quit eating sugar?

Whether nibbling on a late-night piece of cake or topping off on potato chips, sweet food varieties appear to continue to slip into your eating routine. In any event, when on a severe, pre-divided diet, sugar desires keep on pulling at the forefront of your thoughts, directing you on an unending pursuit. To truly beat the desires, you want to figure out them and utilize that comprehension against them.

Sort Out Needing Timings

It might appear to be that your desires are irregular and jump into your head at the most terrible times conceivable. Luckily, desires are entirely planned, making them simpler to battle. When you know the planning of your desires, you can zero in on trigger times and get ready for the fight to come.

To find the exact timing, rehearsing mindfulness is useful. Desires come from your inner mind, so without cognizant mindfulness, you may not understand that you generally wind up looking for a sugar fix simultaneously of day. When you have your times down, you're prepared to begin vanquishing your sugar desires

Remove Sugar

While it may not sound simple, removing sugar from your eating regimen totally can be extremely powerful in quieting desires. Following a week or so of sugar-free dinners and tidbits, the pull of your desires can turn out to be nearly non-existent and a lot more straightforward to disregard.

While going to a social commitment, for example, a birthday celebration or wedding, it very well may be hard to stay away from sugar, as desserts are a cultural standard. A periodic sweet piece of cake may not completely ruin your solid way of life, yet it can get your desires back to full power. Yet again before taking a nibble of a sweet treat, gauge the expense and plan to fight your desires.

Fabricate a Sound Daily Schedule

Irregular abstaining from excessive food intake or sugar fasting isn't sufficient to vanquish your desires. To overcome them, you should execute sound everyday practice in your routine. This could be picking better snacks at the supermarket or going for a run each day. By getting your home free from sugar and keeping your brain and body dynamic consistently, you can start to move your eating routine away from sugar and towards supporting, filling food varieties. With this setup, finding sugar to entice your desires requires making a special effort; more prominent exertion gives normal discouragement from eating sugar.

Not a wide range of sugar is terrible for your well-being, however, to conquer desires, it tends to be useful to remove them all. When the desires for sugar have been hushed, take a stab at exploring different avenues regarding leafy foods containing high measures of fiber close to normal sugars. On the off chance that they don't reestablish their desires, carrying out them into your eating routine is solid and delicious.

Sugar can appear to be all over, and the desire for it can compel you into a way of life you hate. By observing your desires, keeping them from sugar, and concocting an arrangement to keep them calm, you can assume command over your life and eat the way that encourages you.

The subject of how to beat sugar desires is a typical one since a genuine issue a great many people are battling with. Sugar desires are one of the most well-known food desires in the US today, and many individuals are looking for ways of beating it unequivocally.

The typical American consumes around 152 pounds of sugar a year. That is approximately 22 teaspoons every day. Also, youngsters, consume considerably more, at 34 teaspoons each day, which makes almost 1 out of 4 teens prediabetic or type 2 diabetic. This is the reason 70% of Americans and 40% of children are overweight. As per research, 98% of ladies and 68% of men have encountered sugar desires. Also, the more sugar you eat, the more you're probably going to ache for it since sugar is multiple times as habit-forming as cocaine.

It's not difficult to desire sugar when you're anxious, tired, or generally not feeling your best — also that it can cheer you up at the time. In the long haul, be that as it may, unreasonable sugar utilization can prompt weight gain and medical problems like diabetes and coronary illness. In this way, assuming you're needing sugar, the best strategy is to check those desires before they get the better of you.

While there's no enchanted projectile to stop sugar desires, there are a few different ways that can assist you with figuring out how to beat sugar desires and remain focused on your eating routine.

1. Integrate sweet flavors as sugar options

Going for an elective will assist with fooling your brain into imagining that you're having real sugar.

Rather than the typical warm beverages with sugar and syrup, go for sweet flavors, for example, cardamom, coriander, pumpkin pie zest (cinnamon, ginger), and Ceylon cinnamon.

If you seriously love hot cocoa, you can utilize a limited quantity of cocoa powder or unsweetened cocoa blend instead of sugar (I use carob all things considered).

While baking, have a go at adding one teaspoon of ground cinnamon or 1/2 teaspoon of ground ginger per cup of flour called for in your recipe.

These flavors by and large have a better taste however don't contain sugar. At the point when you add them to food sources, you will get that sweet taste, and your psyche will think you are having something sweet when you are not.

2. Trade carbonated drinks for carbonated water

Nothing can beat carbonated water with regards to extinguishing your thirst and controlling sugar desires. Carbonated drinks like pop, sweet tea, and Caffeinated drinks have a ton of sugar and are for the most part not great for you. Nonetheless, it very well may be hard to give up, particularly assuming that you are going to parties or in the late spring when you maintain that something should quiet the intensity.

Assuming that you're attempting to control your sugar desires, you might need to consider supplanting these carbonated drinks with seltzer water (read the mark and ensure there is no added sugar). Note that drinking Seltzer water might conceivably cause gastrointestinal aggravations, such as bulging and gas so you should keep away from it. Rather stick to water, homegrown tea, and lemon water.

Take a stab at imbuing your water with newly pressed natural product juices like lemon or normal spices for an alternate flavour insight. You can likewise incorporate any sweet flavour and add a sprinkle of a normal squeeze, for example, cranberry or cherry juice to give it a tone.

3. Eat entire food sources

In any case, thinking about how to beat sugar desires? Stop handling food sources! Table sugar is concealed in many handled food sources, from sauces and salad dressings to honest bites. While you're attempting to stop sugar hankering, you should avoid sweet food varieties or food sources with added sugars.

Furthermore, if you end up continually needing sugar, change to an eating routine zeroed in on entire food sources all things being equal. The normal supplements found in these sound choices will control your sugar desires. Eating entire food varieties beats sugar desires in various ways. At the point when you eat new food varieties, your body gets various supplements that it can ingest rather than simply void calories. Additionally, because entire food varieties are seriously fulfilling, you'll eat less without a second thought — which is frequently where sugar desires come from in any case. Some exploration has likewise found that individuals who eat generally new products of the soil don't want handled, sweet unhealthy food in any case. So to check sugar desires, begin by eating genuine food! While buying food items available, most people might need to go for sans fat-handled food varieties thinking they are better. In any case, eating entire food varieties containing their regular fat, fiber, and different supplements will assist with controlling desires until your next feast.

4. Keep away from basic carbs

Is it safe to say that you are as yet considering how to beat sugar desires? Stop handling food sources!

Table sugar is concealed in many handled food sources, from sauces and salad dressings to guiltless tidbits. While you're attempting to stop sugar hankering, you really should avoid sweet food sources or food varieties with added sugars. What's more, if you end up continually needing sugar, change to an eating regimen zeroed in on entire food sources all things considered. The regular supplements found in these sound choices will check your sugar desires.

Eating entire food sources beats sugar desires in various ways. At the point when you eat new food varieties, your body gets different supplements that it can retain rather than simply void calories. Likewise, because entire food varieties are fulfilling, you'll eat less without even batting an eye — which is frequently where sugar desires come from in any case. Some exploration has additionally found that individuals who eat generally new products of the soil don't want handled, sweet unhealthy food in any case. Thus, to control sugar desires, begin by eating genuine food!

Straightforward starches like white flour, white pasta, bread, and white potatoes discharge high measures of sugar when processed. This gives you a fast spike in blood glucose, subsequently a speedy increase in energy. However, you'll get a pulverize because these food varieties miss the mark on fibre to support their sugar discharge. The hankering will likewise deteriorate because you're currently desiring a greater amount of the energy you encountered than the actual food.

5. protein and fat with each feast

Protein and fat log jam assimilation, encouraging you longer and checking sugar desires better. Eating on nuts or a little modest bunch of trail blend when your sugar hankering comes the area of strength for on-do ponders. Assuming you should nibble, avoid sweet desserts — it will just exacerbate the situation! Stay with natural products or yogurt. Assuming you should have something sweet, stay with a new or frozen natural product (not canned). You'll get less added sugar that way.

6. Just quit

Albeit the initial not many days can be testing, disposing of any type of straightforward sugars, including counterfeit sugars from your eating routine, can be the most ideal way to move toward your desires. This strategy works best when you have somebody to keep you responsible, essentially toward the start. Be it your mate or companion, find somebody keen on doing likewise and allow it to be a type of challenge, for instance, a ten-day sans sugar challenge.

When you're on the 10th day, your taste buds would have changed, and you would have no desire to return.

7. Remove caffeinated beverages and natural product juices aside from green vegetable juice.

Squeezing takes off all the fiber that could end up being useful to dial back the arrival of sugar, meaning you won't get that fast spike. This likewise implies you'll encounter the other advantages of the natural product. Polishing off natural product juice or caffeinated beverages will cause a spike in glucose, trailed by a radical drop. This is because these beverages have no fiber, so the sugar will rapidly be delivered into the circulation system. This will set off insulin discharge, which will rapidly move glucose out of the blood, causing a drop with a resulting hankering for more sugar.

8. Deal with your pressure

At the point when you're anxious, cortisol goes up, which makes you hungry and ache for sugar.

High-fiber plant-based food varieties like green peas, flaxseed, pistachios, kale, broccoli, almonds, berries, and sesame seeds can assist with decreasing your feelings of anxiety and assist with forestalling desires.

9. Get sufficient rest

Under 8 hours of rest, a day expands your craving chemicals and drives you to indulge. Additionally, a lot of caffeine and liquor can deny you rest.

The best plant-based food sources to assist with improving your rest incorporate chamomile tea, tart cherries, tart cherry juice, seeds, and kiwi.

The fact that something is missing makes craving a decent sign. If you're wanting sugar, it demonstrates various things, including mind molding, mineral lack, blood glucose irregularity, deficient rest, or high feelings of anxiety. So analyze yourself and make that striking stride in handling the singular reasons for your desires. With time the desires will blur off.

10. Pursue solid routines in the first part of the day

One of my #1 ways of checking sugar desires is pursuing solid routines in my mornings. Having a healthy breakfast, getting some activity, and arranging your day all put you in a good position — and make it more straightforward to keep away from undesirable calories later in the day.

CHAPTER 3

The reality with regards to FAT: It's NOT What You Think

For what reason are trans fats awful for you, polyunsaturated and monounsaturated fats great for you, and soaked fats some in the middle between? For a long time, fat was a four-letter word. We were encouraged to oust it from our eating regimens whenever the situation allows. We changed to low-fat food sources. Be that as it may, the shift didn't make us better, presumably because we cut back on sound fat as well as destructive ones.

You might ponder isn't fat terrible for you, however, your body needs some fat from food. It's a significant wellspring of energy. It assists you with retaining a few nutrients and minerals. Fat is expected to assemble cell films, the imperative outside of every cell, and the sheaths encompassing nerves. It is fundamental for blood coagulation, muscle development, and aggravation. For long-haul well-being, a few facts are superior to other people. Great fats incorporate monounsaturated and polyunsaturated fats. Awful ones incorporate modern-made trans fats. Immersed fats fall someplace in the centre.

All fats have a comparative synthetic design: a chain of carbon particles clung to hydrogen molecules. What compels one fat not quite the same as another is the length and state of the carbon chain and the number of hydrogen iotas associated with the carbon particles. Slight contrasts in structure convert into pivotal contrasts in structure and capability.

Awful trans fats

The most horrendously terrible sort of dietary fat is the thoughtful known as trans-fat. It is a result of a cycle called hydrogenation that is utilized to transform sound oils into solids and to keep them from becoming smelly. Trans fats have no realized medical advantages and there is no protected degree of utilization.

From the get-go in the twentieth hundred years, trans fats were tracked down mostly in strong margarine and vegetable shortening. As food producers learned better approaches to utilize to some extent hydrogenated vegetables oils, they started showing up in everything from business treats and baked goods to cheap food French fries. Trans fats are presently restricted in the U.S. furthermore, numerous different nations.

Eating food sources rich in trans fats builds how unsafe LDL cholesterol is in the circulatory system and decreases how valuable HDL cholesterol is. Trans fats make irritation, which is connected to coronary illness, stroke, diabetes, and other persistent circumstances. They add to insulin obstruction, which expands the gamble of creating type 2 diabetes. Indeed, even modest quantities of trans fats can hurt well-being: for each 2% of calories from trans-fat consumed day to day, the gamble of coronary illness ascends by 23%.

In the middle between immersed fats

Immersed fats are normal in the American eating routine. They are strong at room temperature — think cooled bacon oil, however, what is soaked fat? Normal wellsprings of immersed fat incorporate red meat, entire milk and other entire milk dairy food varieties, cheddar, coconut oil, and many industrially pre-arranged heated merchandise and different food varieties.

"Soaked" here alludes to the number of hydrogen molecules encompassing every carbon iota. The chain of carbon molecules holds however many hydrogen iotas as could be expected under the circumstances — it's soaked with hydrogens.

Is soaked fat terrible for you? An eating routine wealthy in soaked fats can drive-up all-out cholesterol, and influence the equilibrium toward more unsafe LDL cholesterol, which prompts blockages to frame in conduits in the heart and somewhere else in the body. Thus, most sustenance specialists prescribe restricting immersed fat to under 10% of calories daily. A small bunch of ongoing reports has ruined the connection between soaked fat and coronary illness. One meta-examination of 21 investigations expressed that there was insufficient proof to infer that soaked fat expands the gamble of coronary illness, yet supplanting immersed fat with polyunsaturated fat may for sure diminish the chance of coronary illness.

Two other significant examinations limited the solution somewhat, presuming that supplanting soaked fat with polyunsaturated fats like vegetable oils or high-fiber sugars is the smartest choice for diminishing the gamble of coronary illness, yet supplanting immersed fat with profoundly handled carbs could do the inverse.

Great monounsaturated and polyunsaturated fats

Great fats come for the most part from vegetables, nuts, seeds, and fish. They contrast with soaked fats by having fewer hydrogen molecules attached to their carbon chains. Sound fats are fluid at room temperature, and not strong. There are two general classifications of useful fats: monounsaturated and polyunsaturated fats.

Monounsaturated fats. At the point when you plunge your bread in olive oil at an Italian eatery, you're getting for the most part monounsaturated fat.

Monounsaturated fats have a solitary carbon-to-carbon twofold security. The outcome is that it has two fewer hydrogen molecules than an immersed fat and a curve at the twofold bond. This design keeps monounsaturated fats fluid at room temperature.

The disclosure that monounsaturated fat could be empowering came from the Seven Nations Study during the 1960s. It uncovered that individuals in Greece and different pieces of the Mediterranean locale partook in a low pace of coronary illness despite a high-fat eating regimen. The fundamental fat in their eating regimen, however, was not the immersed creature fat normal in nations with higher paces of coronary illness. It was olive oil, which contains chiefly monounsaturated fat. This tracking down created a flood of interest in olive oil and the Mediterranean eating regimen," a way of eating viewed as a restorative decision today.

Although there's no suggested everyday admission of monounsaturated fats, the Public Foundation of Medication suggests involving them however much as could be expected alongside polyunsaturated fats to supplant immersed and trans fats.

Polyunsaturated fats. At the point when your empty fluid cooking oil into a skillet, there's a decent opportunity you're utilizing polyunsaturated fat. Corn oil, sunflower oil, and safflower oil are normal models. Polyunsaturated fats are fundamental fats. That implies they're expected for ordinary body capabilities, however, your body can't make them. Along these lines, you should get them from food. Polyunsaturated fats are utilized to fabricate cell films and the cover of nerves. They are required for blood coagulation, muscle development, and irritation.

Polyunsaturated fat has at least two twofold securities in its carbon chain. There are two primary sorts of polyunsaturated fats: omega-3 unsaturated fats and omega-6 unsaturated fats. The numbers allude to the distance between the start of the carbon chain and the primary twofold bond. The two kinds offer medical advantages.

Eating polyunsaturated fats instead of soaked fats or exceptionally refined sugars diminishes unsafe LDL cholesterol and further develops the cholesterol profile. It likewise brings down fatty substances.

Great wellsprings of omega-3 unsaturated fats incorporate greasy fish like salmon, mackerel, sardines, flaxseeds, pecans, canola oil, and un-hydrogenated soybean oil. Food sources rich in linoleic corrosive and other omega-6 unsaturated fats incorporate vegetable oils like safflower, soybean, sunflower, pecan, and corn oils.

The Capability of Fat

Muscle versus fat, or fat tissue, is a perplexing organ. It contains fat cells, nerves, resistant cells, and connective tissue. Its fundamental occupation is to store and deliver energy, contingent upon the body's requirements. Fat answers signals like the chemical insulin, which advises fat tissue to store fat. "There are additionally nerves that go from your cerebrum to your fat and say, 'Hello, we need more energy here. Could you at any point free some fat because different cells in the body need it? Fat tissue is likewise a significant creator of chemicals and substance couriers that speak with tissues and organs all through the body. It's an exemplary endocrine organ, the greatest one in the body. Chemicals created by fat tissue manage digestion and insulin responsiveness. They assist the body with utilizing supplements effectively. For instance, it's the essential maker of adiponectin. This chemical increment insulin responsiveness - something beneficial for holding blood glucose levels under control - and diminishes aggravation. Too little adiponectin can prompt sort 2 diabetes and other metabolic sicknesses.

Another chemical is leptin, which controls craving. "On the off chance that you have no adipocytes [fat cells], you have no leptin. You feel like you have no energy stores and get voraciously eager," Corvera says. Fat tissue likewise delivers different substances that impact aggravation and insusceptible capability.

Various Kinds of Fat Cells

While all fat cells could resemble each other the same from an external perspective, they can have various capabilities, contingent upon their sort. There are three fundamental sorts of fat cells.

• White fat: These are the body's fundamental kind of fat cells. They store energy and produce chemicals like leptin and adiponectin. They are to a great extent tracked down in the chest, gut, and legs.

• Earthy coloured fat: What's special about brown, or thermogenic, fat is that it consumes energy and produces heat in specific circumstances, similar to a chilly climate. Individuals with more earthy-coloured fat will generally be less fatty and better, contrasted with those with less earthy-coloured fat. Concentrates show that earthy-coloured fat further develops digestion and decreases the gamble of infections like sort 2 diabetes, coronary course illness, and hypertension. It's tracked down in the neck, upper chest, shoulder, and stomach.

• Beige fat: at times, white fat changes into "beige" or "brite" fat cells. Like earthy-coloured fat, it consumes energy to deliver heat.

Specialists are concentrating on whether they can tackle the positive characteristics of brown and beige fat and use them to treat stoutness.

Fat additionally acts contrastingly relying upon where it's found: the gut, thigh, or close to your organs. With regards to wellbeing, area matters.

• Instinctive fats: Fat put away somewhere down in the tummy and around organs significantly affects the liver, an organ basic to digestion. It's additionally connected to illnesses like cardiovascular sickness, disease, asthma, and dementia. Blood that leaves instinctive fat goes straightforwardly to the liver and carries with it anything made by the fat tissue, including unsaturated fats, chemicals, and favorable to incendiary synthetic substances. We develop more instinctive fat with age. Fat capacity shifts from the lower body to the tummy, particularly in ladies.

• **Subcutaneous fat**: The fat simply under the skin is the most copious in the body. This sort of fat demonstration diversely relies upon where it's situated, as indicated by Broiled. Subcutaneous tummy fat makes more unsaturated fats, which can increment insulin obstruction and the gamble of metabolic illness. Subcutaneous fat in the lower body, then again, takes up and stores fat proficiently. It's thought of as defensive against sickness.

The amount Is Excessive?

Fat is a fundamental piece of our bodies. Too little or an excess of fat is unfortunate. "You must have the perfect sum," says Seared, however, the perfect sum differs from one individual to another. A significant thought is how much tissue you have access to store fat, which can rely upon your qualities. If you can't make a great deal of fat, you will not have sufficient room to store additional calories. "It will pour out over into your liver, muscles, and heart. That is the very thing that brings about metabolic illness."

As opposed to pondering weight or level of muscle versus fat, think about your waist-to-hip proportion. The research proposes that how fat is conveyed across the body matters more than how much muscle-to-fat ratio is with regards to by and large well-being.

To get your midriff to-hip proportion, utilize a measuring tape to quantify your midsection and hips in centimeters. Partition your abdomen estimation by your hip estimation. The World Wellbeing Association says that the gamble of medical problems is more noteworthy for men who have a midriff to-hip proportion of 0.90 or higher, and for ladies with a midsection to-hip proportion of 0.85 centimeters or higher.

You can likewise actually look at your abdomen boundary. The possibilities of medical issues connected with weight are higher for men with a midriff of more than 40 inches, and for (a pregnant) lady) with a midsection circuit of more than 35 inches, as per the CDC.

"Individuals understood that midriff size is a gamble factor for type 2 diabetes, other ongoing infection, and, surprisingly, sudden passing," Seared says. Alternately, having more muscle versus fat in your lower body might assist with safeguarding your well-being. Research likewise proposes that fat acts contrastingly in ladies and men. In one review, higher bulk appeared to safeguard ladies and men from cardiovascular illness. However, ladies with higher fat, paying little mind to bulk, were more averse to passing on from coronary illness - yet provided that their pulse, glucose, and cholesterol were taken care of. (Whether they were taking chemical swap treatment for menopausal side effects likewise made a difference.).

Muscle versus fat isn't just about your size or what you look like. What is important is what it means for your well-being. You must have solid fat tissue to be sound in any remaining parts of your physical and psychological well-being.

Heart wellbeing

Some proof recommends that monounsaturated fats can further develop heart well-being.

For instance, the allowed concentrate demonstrated a connection between admissions of MUFAs and polyunsaturated unsaturated fats (PUFAs) and a lower chance of cardiovascular illness.

The AHA likewise prompts that monounsaturated fats can further develop somebody's cholesterol profile and lower their gamble of coronary illness and stroke. They add that monounsaturated fats likewise contribute to the cell reinforcement of vitamin E in the eating routine, which many individuals living in the US are lacking in.A survey makes sense of that contrasted with eating a high soaked fat feast, consuming a high monounsaturated fat dinner has the accompanying advantages:

• bigger, lighter low-thickness lipoprotein (LDL) particles, which are less risky to heart wellbeing
• quicker leeway of fats in the wake of eating
• more fat consuming and less fat stockpiling
• decrease in fasting fatty oils and coagulation factors

Also, 2019 surveys on human veins showed that MUFAs forestalled the harmful impacts of soaked fats on cells.

Although researchers need to do more research, the specialists propose that the defensive impacts of MUFAs could be significant for heart well-being.

Diabetes

As per a 2016 fundamental survey on meta-examination, slims down high in MUFAs might help individuals with type 2 diabetes.

The audit recommended that contrasted with high starch eats less, high MUFA counts calories diminished the accompanying gamble factors:

• fasting plasma glucose
• fatty substances
• body weight
• systolic circulatory strain

The specialists additionally found that high MUFA consumes fewer calories expanding valuable high-thickness lipoprotein (HDL) cholesterol.Furthermore, high MUFA abstains from food meaningfully affected fasting glucose more than high polyunsaturated unsaturated fat weight control plans.

Aggravation and corpulence

As per a 2021 survey, proof connects MUFAs to calming states and less corpulence. Then again, soaked fats are incendiary and can add to abundance weight and corpulence.

The specialists bring up that the Mediterranean eating routine incorporates 60% MUFAs contrasted and 36% in the Western eating regimen.

Individuals consuming a Mediterranean eating routine have less occurrence of heftiness and its connected fiery impacts, like a cardiovascular infection.

Besides, the TOMORROW study recommended that mitigating MUFAs could stifle sickness action in patients with rheumatoid joint pain.

Wellsprings of monounsaturated fat

Albeit creature items, for example, eggs and meat contain MUFAs, the most extravagant sources are plant food sources. Great wellsprings of MUFAs include:

- olive oil
- canola oil
- nut oil
- sesame oil
- safflower oil
- avocados

- peanut butter
- nuts and seeds

CHAPTER 4

THE Genuine Reason for Coronary illness

To comprehend the reasons for coronary illness, might assist with understanding how the heart functions.
- The heart is separated into chambers — two upper chambers (atria) and two lower chambers (ventricles).
- The right half of the heart moves blood to the lungs through veins (pneumonic courses).
- In the lungs, blood gets oxygen and afterward gets back to the left half of the heart through the aspiratory veins.
- The left half of the heart then, at that point, siphons the blood through the aorta and out to the remainder of the body.
Heart valves
Four heart valves — the aortic, mitral, pneumonic, and tricuspid — keep the blood moving the correct way. The valves open just a single way and just as needs be. Valves should open as far as possible and close firmly so there's no spillage.
Pulses

A thumping heart presses (contracts) and loosens up in a nonstop cycle.
• During withdrawal (systole), the lower heart chambers (ventricles) press tight. This activity powers blood to the lungs and the remainder of the body.
• During unwinding (diastole), the ventricles load up with blood from the upper heart chambers (atria).

Electrical framework

The heart's electrical framework keeps it pulsating. The heartbeat controls the consistent trade of oxygen-rich blood with oxygen-unfortunate blood. This trade keeps you alive.
• Electrical signs start in the upper right chamber (right chamber).
• The signs make a trip through particular pathways to the lower heart chambers (ventricles). This advises the heart to siphon.

Coronary illness alludes to any condition influencing the cardiovascular framework. There are a few unique sorts of coronary illnesses, and they influence the heart and veins in various ways.

The areas underneath check out a few distinct kinds of coronary illness in more detail.

Coronary supply route illness

Coronary supply route illness, otherwise called coronary illness, is the most widely recognized sort of coronary illness.

It creates when the conduits that supply blood to the heart become obstructed with plaque. This makes them solidify and limit. Plaque contains cholesterol and different substances.

Subsequently, the blood supply diminishes, and the heart gets less oxygen and fewer supplements. In time, the heart muscle debilitates, and there is a gamble of cardiovascular breakdown and arrhythmias.

The point when plaque develops in the courses is called arthrosis Plaque in the conduits can burst from blockages and cause the bloodstream to stop, which can prompt a coronary episode.

Inherent heart abandons

An individual with an inherent heart deformity is brought into the world with a heart issue. There are many kinds of innate heart defects, including:

• Abnormal heart valves: Valves may not open as expected, or they might spill blood.

• Septal imperfections: There is an opening in the wall between either the lower chambers or the upper offices of the heart.

• Atresia: One of the heart valves is absent.

Inherent coronary illness can include major primary issues, like the shortfall of a ventricle or issues with uncommon associations between the principal corridors that leave the heart.

Numerous inherent heart surrenders cause no recognizable side effects and just become clear during a standard clinical check.

As per the America Heart Affiliation, heart mumbles frequently influence youngsters, yet just an area because of a deformity.

Arrhythmia

Arrhythmia alludes to a sporadic heartbeat. It happens when the electrical motivations that coordinate the heartbeat don't work accurately. Subsequently, the heart might pulsate excessively fast, too leisurely, or whimsically.

There are different kinds of arrhythmias, including:

• Tachycardia: This alludes to a fast heartbeat.

• Bradycardia: This alludes to a sluggish heartbeat.

• Untimely withdrawals: This alludes to an early heartbeat.

• Atrial fibrillation: This is a kind of unpredictable heartbeat.

An individual might see an inclination like a vacillating or a dashing heart.

Now and again, arrhythmias can be dangerous or have extreme entanglements.

Enlarged cardiomyopathy

In enlarged cardiomyopathy, the heart chambers become widened, implying that the heart muscle extends and becomes slenderer. The most well-known reasons for enlarged cardiomyopathy are past cardiovascular failures, arrhythmias, and poisons, however, hereditary qualities can likewise assume a part.

Thus, the heart becomes more fragile and can't siphon blood as expected. It can bring about arrhythmia, blood clumps in the heart, and cardiovascular breakdown. It generally influences individuals aged 20-60, as per the AHA.

Myocardial localized necrosis

Otherwise called respiratory failure, myocardial localized necrosis includes an interference of the bloodstream to the heart. This can harm or annihilate a piece of the heart muscle.

The most well-known reason for cardiovascular failure is plaque, blood coagulation, or both in a coronary conduit. It can likewise happen if a course unexpectedly limits or fits.

Cardiovascular breakdown

At the point when an individual has a cardiovascular breakdown, their heart is as yet working but not as well as it ought to be. The congestive cardiovascular breakdown is a kind of cardiovascular breakdown that can happen from issues with the siphoning or loosening up capability.

The cardiovascular breakdown can result from untreated coronary corridor sickness, hypertension, arrhythmias, and different circumstances. These circumstances can influence the heart's capacity to siphon or unwind appropriately.

The cardiovascular breakdown can be perilous, yet looking for early treatment for heart-related conditions can assist with forestalling complexities.

Hypertrophic cardiomyopathy

This condition ordinarily creates when a hereditary issue influences the heart muscle. It will in general be an acquired condition.

The walls of the muscle thicken, and withdrawals become more enthusiastic. This influences the heart's capacity to take in and siphon out blood. Now and again, a block can happen.

There might be no side effects, and many individuals don't get a determination. Notwithstanding, hypertrophic cardiomyopathy can demolish over the long run and lead to different heart issues.

Anybody with a family background of this condition ought to request a screening, as getting treatment can assist with forestalling entanglements.

Hypertrophic cardiomyopathy is the primary driver of heart demise among youngsters and competitors under 35 years of age, as per the AHA.

Mitral valve spewing forth

This occasion happens when the mitral valve in the heart doesn't close firmly enough and permits blood to stream once again into the heart.

Thus, blood can't travel through the heart or body effectively, and it can come down to the offices of the heart. In time, the heart can become amplified, and cardiovascular breakdown can result.

Mitral valve prolapses

This happens when the valve folds of the mitral valve don't close as expected. All things considered; they swell into the left chamber. This can cause a heart to mumble.

Mitral valve prolapse isn't generally dangerous, however, certain individuals might have to get treatment for it.

Hereditary variables and connective tissue issues can cause this condition, which influences around 2% of the populace.

Aortic stenosis

In aortic stenosis, the aspiratory valve is thick or combined and doesn't open accurately. This makes it difficult for the heart to siphon blood from the left ventricle into the aorta.

An individual might be brought into the world with it because of intrinsic peculiarities of the valve, or it might foster over the long haul because of calcium stores or scarring.

Side effects

The side effects of coronary illness rely upon the particular kind an individual has. Likewise, some heart conditions cause no side effects by any means.

All things considered; the accompanying side effects might show a heart issue:

• angina, or chest torment

• trouble relaxing

• weakness and discombobulation

• enlarging because of liquid maintenance, or noema

In kids, the side effects of an intrinsic heart imperfection might incorporate cyanosis or a blue hint to the skin, and powerlessness to work out.

A few signs and side effects that could demonstrate cardiovascular failure include:

• chest torment

• windedness

• hearts palpitations

- sickness
- stomach torment
- perspiring
- arm, jaw, back, or leg torment
- a gagging sensation
- enlarged lower legs
- exhaustion
- a sporadic heartbeat

The coronary episode can prompt heart failure, which is the point at which the heart stops and the body can never again work. An individual requires quick clinical consideration on the off chance that they have any side effects of a cardiovascular failure.

Assuming heart failure happens, the individual will require:

- prompt clinical assistance (call 911)
- prompt cardiopulmonary revival
- a shock from a mechanized outside defibrillator, if accessible

Causes and chance variables

Coronary illness creates when there are:

- harm to all or part of the heart
- an issue with the veins prompting or from the heart
- a low stock of oxygen and supplements to the heart
- an issue with the beat of the heart

At times, there is a hereditary reason. In any case, some way of life variables and ailments can likewise build the gamble. These include:

- hypertension
- elevated cholesterol

- smoking
- a high admission of liquor
- overweight and heftiness
- diabetes
- a family background of coronary illness
- dietary decisions
- age
- a background marked by toxemia during pregnancy
- low movement levels
- rest aponia
- high pressure and tension levels
- broken heart valves

The World Wellbeing Association refers to neediness and stress as two key elements adding to a worldwide expansion in heart and cardiovascular illness

CHAPTER 5

Past THE MEDITERRANEAN Eating regimen: WHAT DO I EAT

What is the Mediterranean Eating routine?
The Mediterranean Eating routine is an approach to eating that underscores plant-based food sources and healthy fats.
As a rule, if you follow a Mediterranean Eating routine, you'll eat:
• Bunches of vegetables, natural products, beans, lentils, and nuts.
• Loads of entire grains, similar to entire wheat bread and earthy-colored rice.
• A lot of additional virgin olive oil (EVOO) as a wellspring of solid fat.
• A moderate measure of fish, particularly fish wealthy in omega-3 unsaturated fat.
• A moderate measure of cheddar and yogurt.
• Almost no meat, picking poultry rather than red meat.
• Almost no desserts, sweet beverages, or spread.
• A moderate measure of wine with dinners (yet if you don't as of now drink, don't begin).
A dietitian can assist you with changing this eating routine case by case in light of your clinical history, hidden conditions, sensitivities, and inclinations.

What is the meaning of the Mediterranean Eating regimen?

There are numerous meanings of the eating routine (each with marginally various objectives for servings). That is because the eating regimen centers around by and large eating designs as opposed to severe equations or estimations. It's likewise founded on eating designs across a wide range of Mediterranean nations, each with its subtleties. Since there's no single definition, the Mediterranean Eating regimen is adaptable, and you can fit it into your necessities.

What are the advantages of the Mediterranean Eating regimen?

The Mediterranean Eating routine has many advantages, including:

• Bringing down your gamble of cardiovascular infection.

• Supporting a body weight that is smart for you.

• Supporting solid glucose, circulatory strain, and cholesterol.

• Bringing down your gamble of metabolic disorders.

• Supporting a good arrangement of stomach microbiota (microscopic organisms and different microorganisms) in your stomach-related framework.

• Bringing down your gamble for specific sorts of diseases.

• Easing back the decay of cerebrum capability as you age.

• Assisting you with living longer.

Cardiologists frequently suggest the Mediterranean Eating regimen because broad examination upholds its heart-sound advantages. One review checked out individuals at high gamble of cardiovascular illness for more than five years. These individuals were parted into two gatherings. One gathering followed the Mediterranean Eating routine, and the other gathering followed a low-fat eating routine. The Mediterranean Eating regimen bunch had a 30% lower relative gamble of cardiovascular occasions contrasted with the low-fat eating routine gathering. Such occasions included coronary episodes, stroke, or cardiovascular-related passing.

Specialists accept these defensive advantages are part of the way because of the sound fats you eat with the Mediterranean Eating regimen. These come from food sources like olive oil, nuts, and fish.

For what reason is the Mediterranean Eating regimen great for me?

The Mediterranean Eating regimen incorporates various supplements that cooperate to help your body. There's no single food or fix answerable for the Mediterranean Eating routine's advantages. All things being equal, the eating routine is great for you in light of the mix of supplements it gives.

Consider an ensemble with many individuals singing. A single voice could keep part of the melody; however, you want every one of the voices to meet up to accomplish the full impact. Additionally, the Mediterranean Eating regimen works by providing you with an ideal mix of supplements that blend to help your well-being.

There are not many weight controls plans as generally suggested by specialists as the Mediterranean eating routine. That is because it's not exactly an eating regimen by any means — it's a way of life, says Elena Paravantes-Hargitt, an enlisted dietitian-nutritionist who spends significant time in the Mediterranean eating routine and is the pioneer behind Olive Tomato. Paravantes-Hargitt lives in Greece. "It depends on how individuals in specific pieces of the Mediterranean were living and eating, so it is very manageable and sensible," she says.

It's likewise difficult to look past these numbers concerning your ticker. In an investigation of almost 26,000 ladies, those with the most elevated adherence to the Mediterranean eating routine depended 28% less inclined to foster coronary illness.

The eating routine might be especially defensive since it can diminish aggravation. In addition, the cell reinforcement compound called hydroxytyrosol, found in food varieties that are signs of the eating routine (organic products, nuts, extra-virgin olive oil), has been displayed to fix heart-hurting free extreme harm, the creators say.

While living longer and dealing with your heart are critical to you, there's no rejecting that you might be keen on the Mediterranean eating routine for its weight reduction potential. Albeit not a principal objective of this eating approach, it might assist with balancing out your weight — without causing you to feel denied. A concentrate by scientists at Harvard College and Emory College followed a gathering of overweight or large grown-ups on the Mediterranean eating routine and a benchmark group eating a standard American eating regimen enhanced with fish oil, pecans, and grape juice — food sources that supply key supplements in the Mediterranean eating routine — for quite some time.

A standard American eating routine is wealthy in food sources that are high in soaked fat, added sugar, and salt. Contrasted and the benchmark group, Mediterranean eating regimen supporters lost more weight, decreased their blood levels of incendiary markers, and brought down their absolute cholesterol and LDL ("awful") cholesterol. The reward: It shouldn't have been a weight reduction concentrate regardless (that was only a pleasant reward) so the two gatherings ate a comparative number of calories.

Concerning gambles, dietitians frequently prescribe a Mediterranean-style diet to those overseeing constant infections like sort 2 diabetes. While this diet is viewed as heart-sound, the American Heart Affiliation calls attention to that it contains more fat than is commonly suggested (however it's low in undesirable soaked fat).

The primary focus point: This is perhaps the best way you can eat, yet like all the other things, if you're changing your eating regimen or involving an eating routine in your treatment plan for an illness, consistently converse with your PCP first.

5 Ways to Make Your Mediterranean Eating routine Arrangement

Fortunately, because this is a way of eating versus a bunch of inflexible standards, you can completely tweak this way to deal with suit your preferences. There's no following this perfectly or tumbling off the cart and feeling like a disappointment. "Indeed, even inside the Mediterranean eating regimen there are what we call 'unique event days' where you might eat more or eat food sources that maybe are not exceptionally sound, yet that is entire of the way of life," Paravantes-Hargitt says. "Food is to be delighted in, and the Mediterranean eating routine advances a solid relationship with food. 'Cheating' is important for the Mediterranean eating routine. You simply proceed with the following day as though nothing occurred."

In any case, the following are five significant hints to kick you off:

1. Eat more vegetables. In addition to the fact that they are a staple that you're likely not eating enough of at any rate yet they're spending plan cordial and proposition a large group of wholesome advantages, says Paravantes-Hargitt, for example, being high in fiber and protein, low in fat, and a wellspring of B nutrients, iron, and cell reinforcements. These incorporate lentils, dried peas, beans, and chickpeas (like hummus).

2. Don't exaggerate liquor. One normal misconception is that those following the Mediterranean eating routine beverage a ton of red wine. "The wine polished off

inside the Mediterranean eating routine is finished with some restraint and is constantly drunk with food," Paravantes-Hargitt says. "Generally, a modest quantity of wine, around 3 to 4 ounces, would be polished off with the feast."

3. Make meat a side. Customarily, individuals ate meat just for extraordinary events, like a Sunday dinner, and, surprisingly, then, in modest quantities, says Paravantes-Hargitt. Attempt to integrate more veggie-lover-based mains, for example, those revolving around beans, tofu, or seitan, into your day. "A decent spot to begin is going veggie lover one day seven days," she says. At the point when you do eat meat, center around decisions like skinless chicken and save red meat for one time each week or two times every month.

4. Eat fewer desserts. Very much like meat, make sweets an exceptional event dish. That doesn't mean sugar is out — have a piece in your espresso if you'd like, for example, "however consistently, there isn't a lot of sugar eaten," says Paravantes-Hargitt.

5. Cook with olive oil. Make extra-virgin olive oil the oil you cook with. While getting carried away with this oil can prompt weight gain (it's fat all things considered, so the calories can add up rapidly), it's wealthy in heart-solid polyunsaturated and monounsaturated fat, so you can feel better about keeping a container convenient in the kitchen. You can likewise involve it in cool applications to make salad dressing or to sprinkle on cooked veggies or side dishes.

Likely advantages

The Mediterranean eating routine has been connected to an extensive rundown of medical advantages.
Advances heart wellbeing

The Mediterranean eating regimen has been read widely for its capacity to advance heart well-being.
Research shows that the Mediterranean eating routine might try and be connected to a lower chance of coronary illness and stroke. One review looked at the impacts of the Mediterranean eating routine and a low-fat eating routine and revealed that the Mediterranean eating routine was more compelling at easing back the movement of plaque developed in the conduits, which is a significant gamble factor for coronary illness.
 Another examination demonstrates the way that the Mediterranean eating routine could likewise assist with bringing down degrees of diastolic and systolic circulatory strain to help heart well-being.

Upholds sound glucose levels

The Mediterranean eating regimen energizes different supplements and thick food varieties, including organic products, vegetables, nuts, seeds, entire grains, and heart-sound fats. Thusly, following this eating example might assist with settling glucose levels and safeguard against type 2 diabetes.
Curiously, various investigations have discovered that the Mediterranean eating routine can lessen fasting

glucose levels and further develop levels of hemoglobin A1C, a marker used to gauge long-haul glucose control. The Mediterranean eating routine has likewise been displayed to diminish insulin opposition, a condition that disables the body's capacity to utilize insulin to direct glucose levels.

Safeguards mind capability

A few investigations show that the Mediterranean eating routine could be helpful for cerebrum well-being and may try and safeguard against mental degradation as you progress in years. For instance, one review including 512 individuals observed that more prominent adherence to the Mediterranean eating regimen was related to further developed memory and decreases in a few gamble factors for Alzheimer's sickness. Another examination has found that the Mediterranean eating regimen might be attached to a lower chance of dementia, mental debilitation, and Alzheimer's illness. Likewise, one enormous survey additionally showed that following the Mediterranean eating routine was connected to upgrades in mental capability, memory, consideration, and handling speed in sound more seasoned grown-ups

For instance, one review including 512 individuals observed that more noteworthy adherence to the Mediterranean eating regimen was related to further developed memory and decreases in a few gamble factors for Alzheimer's illness.

Another examination has found that the Mediterranean eating routine might be attached to a lower chance of dementia, mental debilitation, and Alzheimer's sickness. Additionally, one enormous audit likewise showed that following the Mediterranean eating routine was connected to upgrades in mental capability, memory, consideration, and handling speed in solid more established grown-ups

Food sources to eat on the Mediterranean eating regimen

Remember that the Mediterranean eating regimen addresses a culture similar to cooking, so there's no need to focus on what's permitted or kept away from. Before it was a "diet," MD was only the way that individuals who live close to the Mediterranean ate — individuals who depended on occasional food sources and expected to mind their financial plans and their family's well-being simultaneously, so it's acceptable for you to floor their lead and incorporate as numerous or barely any Mediterranean food varieties as you can. Antiquated grains, such as quinoa, are important for the Mediterranean eating routine. Getty Pictures

That being said, these are the focal food sources in the Mediterranean eating regimen:

• Fish — particularly salmon, sardines, and fish
• New produce — utilize what's privately developed to guarantee newness
• Solid fats — like nuts, avocado, and olive oil
• Lean dairy — like cheddar, Greek yogurt, and milk

• Entire grains — attempt cereals, earthy colored rice, and entire wheat pasta or old grains like quinoa, chia, amaranth, bulgur, and buckwheat

• Wine — with some restraint

The Mediterranean eating regimen food pyramid

The Mediterranean food pyramid offers an extraordinary method for understanding how to ponder your food as opposed to giving you unbending guidelines. It's coordinated by how frequently you ought to remember a food classification for your eating routine, with the food varieties you ought to incorporate most frequently at the base and the food varieties you ought to incorporate less frequently at the top.

The Mediterranean eating routine food pyramid. Getty Pictures

Here is the Mediterranean food pyramid, from base to top:

• Natural products, vegetables, grains (generally entire), olive oil, beans, nuts, vegetables and seeds, spices, and flavors: Consume these at each feast.

• Fish and fish: Eat something like two times every week.

• Poultry, eggs, cheddar, and yogurt: Eat in moderate sums, day to day to week by week, contingent upon the food.

• Meats and desserts: Eat these just infrequently.

Mediterranean Chickpea Salad. TODAY

Food sources to stay away from on the Mediterranean eating routine

There are no completely illegal food varieties on the Mediterranean eating regimen. In any case, you by and large need to adhere to eating food varieties with conspicuous non-logical names. A basic guideline of thumb is that the vast majority of the things you eat shouldn't come in boxes.

Here are a few food varieties to stay away from on the Mediterranean eating routine:

• Liquor (other than wine)

• Spread

• Intensely handled food — like frozen feasts with added sodium, pop, high-sugar refreshments, candy, and handled cheddar

• Handled red meats — like franks, hotdogs, bacon, and lunch meats

• Refined grains — like white bread, white pasta, or anything with white flour

• Refined or handled oils — like soybean oil, safflower oil, corn oil, vegetable oil, canola oil, and any hydrogenated or somewhat hydrogenated oils

Mediterranean eating regimen recipes

• Mediterranean chickpea salad

• Barbecued Mediterranean chicken

• Mediterranean eggplant sandwiches

• Mediterranean heated pasta

• Sheet skillet Greek shrimp

CHAPTER 6

Drug: Enhancements and Solid living that help the heart

The supplement can help your bones, your muscles, and numerous different pieces of your body. And your heart? Research shows that some of them might assist with bringing down cholesterol, further developing pulse, and different things that put you in danger of coronary illness. It's indistinct, however, if they assist with forestalling coronary episodes, strokes, and different issues.

These supplements can be a decent expansion to your heart-solid way of life.

Our cutting-edge world can bring overpowering measures of data pointed toward assisting us with getting better through supplements. Frequently, certain individuals will see enhancements, while others will not. Here are a few enhancements that can assist with helping the impact of a solid eating routine and exercise for your valuable heart, and one enhancement to stay away from.

On the planet, dietary enhancement is substances you eat or drink. They can be nutrients, minerals, spices or different plants, amino acids (the singular structure blocks of protein), or portions of these substances. They can be in pill, case, tablet, or fluid structure. They supplement (add to) the eating routine and ought not to be viewed as a substitute for food.

A few spices and enhancements might help in battling atherosclerosis, the fundamental reason for most coronary illnesses. Atherosclerosis makes plaque develop in your veins, hindering the progression of oxygen-rich blood to your heart and different organs. It can cause a coronary episode and even pass. Atherosclerosis is normal in the created world, yet essentially obscure beyond it, because of the various weight control plans and ways of life of individuals in the created scene.

With such countless enhancements professing to help heart well-being, you might contemplate whether any of them give any advantage. There has been research on the effect of numerous dietary enhancements on cardiovascular well-being. Nonetheless, the outcomes are much of the time not satisfactory since individuals who are bound to utilize dietary enhancements are likewise bound to have better-eating regimens and way of life ways of behaving.

More exploration is expected to verify or refute the job that dietary enhancements might play in heart well-being if any. Until we know more, nutrients and enhancements ought to just be taken under the oversight of a medical care supplier alongside a heart-sound way of life, and not as an essential treatment for heart well-being.

Research shows that a few enhancements might bring down the gamble of coronary illness, while others might hurt those with coronary illness risk factors. Furthermore, a few enhancements may not cause damage but will not give a lot of good for heart well-being all things considered.

A few Enhancement AND Drug THAT HELPS THE HEART

1. Multivitamins and mineral

Nutrients and minerals taken in proper dosages might help with bringing down coronary illness risk. Entire food sources ought to be the primary wellspring of supplements, and examinations show that many individuals miss the mark concerning suggested admissions.

An enhancement can't compensate for unfortunate dietary patterns, yet at times even individuals who have good dieting propensities find it hard to get every one of the natural products, vegetables, and other quality food varieties they need. An enhancement can assist with filling in the holes.

Various investigations propose a positive relationship between taking nutrient and mineral enhancements, and coronary illness anticipation. Nutrient and mineral enhancements can be protected and reasonable and may give a medical advantage.

2. Coenzyme Q10 (Co Q10)

Coenzyme Q10 (CoQ10) is a substance like a nutrient. It is tracked down in each cell of the body. Your body makes CoQ10, and your cells use it to deliver the energy your body needs for cell development and upkeep. It additionally works as a cell reinforcement, which safeguards the body from harm brought about by unsafe atoms. CoQ10 is normally present in limited quantities in a wide assortment of food varieties, however, levels are especially high in organ meats like heart, liver, and kidney, as well as hamburger, soy oil, sardines, mackerel, and peanuts.

Coenzymes assist proteins in attempting to assist with safeguarding the heart and skeletal muscles.

CoQ10 is additionally said to help cardiovascular breakdown, as well as lift energy, and speed recuperation from work out. Certain individuals take it to assist with decreasing the impacts specific drugs can have on the heart, muscles, and different organs.

3. Fibre

The most ideal way to get fibre is from food. In any case, if you do exclude sufficient fibre-rich food from your eating regimen and decide to utilize a fibre supplement, pick an item that has various kinds of fibre in it-both dissolvable and insoluble. While taking a fibre supplement, make certain to remain very much hydrated.

Psyllium fibre might assist with bringing down cholesterol when utilized along with an eating regimen low in cholesterol and immersed fat.

If you decide to take a fibre supplement, be certain you don't coincidentally buy a purgative enhancement all things being equal. The names on the two sorts of enhancements might offer something like "manages inside designs."

Fibre is by all accounts most really utilized related to counting calories and exercise for adding to weight reduction.

4. Omega-3 unsaturated fats

Omega-3 polyunsaturated unsaturated fats are tracked down in oil from specific kinds of fish, vegetables, and other plant sources. These unsaturated fats are not made by the body and should be consumed in the eating regimen or through supplements, frequently "fish oil." Omega-3 polyunsaturated unsaturated fats work by bringing down the body's creation of fatty oils. Elevated degrees of fatty substances can prompt coronary supply route infection, coronary illness, and stroke. Omega-3 polyunsaturated unsaturated fats utilized along with diet and exercise assist with bringing down fatty substance levels in the blood.

In a twofold visually impaired investigation of patients with ongoing cardiovascular breakdown, supplementation with fish oil brought about a little however measurably critical diminishing in the number of patients who passed on or were hospitalized for cardiovascular reasons. In another twofold visually impaired preliminary, supplementation further developed heart capability and diminished the number of hospitalizations in certain patients.

5. Magnesium

Low magnesium levels can be an indicator of coronary illness, research has uncovered. Low magnesium has been connected with cardiovascular gamble factors, for example, hypertension, blood vessel plaque development, calcification of delicate tissues, cholesterol, and solidifying of the corridors.

Magnesium supplements come in different structures and mineral mixes, for example, magnesium citrate, magnesium gluconate, magnesium hydroxide, and the famous type of magnesium sulphate, otherwise called Epsom salt, utilized in showers and foot douses for sore, tired muscles.

Patients with kidney illness should be wary of magnesium, cautions Sherri Rutherford, DO, PeaceHealth Southwest Washington integrative medication, and talk with their primary care physician.

6. L-Carnitine

L-carnitine is an amino corrosive expected to ship fats into the mitochondria (the spot in the cell where fats are transformed into energy). Satisfactory energy creation is fundamental for typical heart capability.

A few examinations involving L-carnitine showed an improvement in heart capability and a decrease in the side effects of angina.

Individuals with congestive cardiovascular breakdown have inadequate oxygenation of the heart, which can harm the heart muscle. Such harm might be decreased by taking L-carnitine supplements.

Taking L-carnitine may likewise assist with diminishing harm and intricacies following a coronary episode.

7. Green tea

Green tea has been delighted in for quite a long time and utilized as a probable powerful guide in treating elevated cholesterol. Green tea has been displayed to bring down complete cholesterol and LDL cholesterol levels as indicated by a few primers and controlled preliminaries. Dr. Rutherford suggests three cups each day, instead of concentrating, since tainting can be a worry as an enhancement.

8. Garlic

Other than making food taste great for some individuals, garlic has been taken orally as an enhancement and has been utilized as a conceivably powerful guide in treating hypertension and coronary supply route sickness.

Garlic can influence blood-coagulating and may expand your gamble of dying. On the off chance that you want a medical procedure, dental work, or an operation, quit taking garlic something like fourteen days early.

9. Nutrient K2

At the point when you catch wind of vitamin K, you might consider the thoughtfulness found in dull salad greens that assists with blood coagulation. That is nutrient K1.

Nutrient K2 is altogether unique. Not at all like nutrient K1, nutrient K2 is found in grass took care of meats and dairy, natto (matured soy), and egg yolks. It works like a "calcium chief" in your body, enacting chemicals that coax calcium out of corridor walls, where its presence is related to an expanded gamble of coronary illness, and into your bones and teeth - where it's required most. Individuals who eat more nutrient K2 are displayed to have a lower hazard of coronary illness, yet most

Western weight control plans miss the mark. It's presumably simplest to get a reliable wellspring of Nutrient K2 from an enhancement that gives 100-200 mcg day to day, taken with dinner.